Frequentl

all about
grape seed
extract

DALLAS CLOUATRE, PhD

AVERY PUBLISHING GROUP

Garden City Park • New York

The information contained in this book is based upon the research and personal and professional experiences of the author. They are not intended as a substitute for consulting with your physician or other health care provider. Any attempt to diagnose and treat an illness should be done under the direction of a health care professional.

The publisher does not advocate the use of any particular health care protocol, but believes the information in this book should be available to the public. The publisher and author are not responsible for any adverse effects or consequences resulting from the use of any of the suggestions, preparations, or procedures discussed in this book. Should the reader have any questions concerning the appropriateness of any procedure or preparation mentioned, the author and the publisher strongly suggest consulting a professional health care advisor.

Series cover designer: Eric Macaluso
Cover image courtesy of PhotoDisk

ISBN: 0-89529-907-0

Copyright © 1998 by Dallas Clouatre, Ph.D.

All rights reserved. No part of this publication may be reproduced, stored in a retrieval system, or transmitted, in any form or by any means, electronic, mechanical, photocopying, recording or otherwise, without the prior written permission of the copyright owner.

Printed in the United States of America

10   9   8   7   6   5   4   3   2

Contents

Introduction

They call it the French Paradox: French people are well known for their love of rich foods—butter, cheese, eggs, sauces—and a diet that contains more saturated fat and cholesterol than is found in the American diet. Yet the French have a heart disease rate that is only about 40 percent of that in the United States.

Why should this be? Ever since the French Paradox was first observed in 1979, scientists have been searching for the reason. One focus of their research: wine, especially red wine, which the French so love and consume as a matter of course with their meals. And sure enough, one study found that people who consumed three to five glasses of wine daily over a twelve-year period had only half the risk of dying of heart disease as compared with those who did not drink wine.

But what about the wine could have this effect? Researchers turned their attention to the grapes from which wine is made. They found substances in grape skins that acted as powerful antioxidants. But the most exciting studies reported that there was a concentration of compounds with health-promoting potential in the seeds of the grapes.

Today, grape seed extract is available in pharmacies and health-food stores across the country. Unfortunately, relatively few Americans are aware of the impressive health potential of grape seed extract and of the bioactive components it contains. *All About Grape Seed Extract* will tell you everything you need to know about this amazing supplement. It starts by answering your basic questions about what it is and how it was discovered. Subsequent chapters detail the benefits that grape seed extract offers for the treatment and/or prevention of conditions as varied as allergies, arthritis, hemorrhoids, night blindness, diabetic retinopathy, premenstrual syndrome (PMS), ulcers, delcining brain function, heart attack, stroke, cancer, hardening of the arteries—even wrinkling of the skin. Finally, there is a chapter explaining how to incorporate grape seed extract into your life. There is even a glossary to help you understand new terms and a reference list of books you might explore for further information. *All About Grape Seed Extract* will give you all the information you need to take advantage of this exciting new supplement.

1.

Grape Seed Extract: An Overview

The notion that good wine promotes good health goes back many centuries. Yet many people were surprised when, in 1979, researchers broke the news that people who lived in countries where wine was a regular accompaniment to meals had a lower incidence of heart attacks and other health problems than people who drank no alcoholic beverages at all. Since then, we have begun to uncover many of the reasons for wine's beneficial effects. And with modern extraction techniques, scientists have been able to give us a natural nutritional supplement that concentrates many of the benefits of red wine. This is grape seed extract. In this chapter, we will look at what exactly grape seed is, how it was discovered, and what makes it offer so many important benefits for health.

Q. Why should I be interested in grape seed extract?

A. Very few items in the nutritional arsenal can boast as many and varied potential benefits as grape seed extract can. Its most important applications are in the areas of allergies, arthritis, diabetes, heart and blood-vessel disorders, and vision problems. It may also have benefits for the healing of wounds and injuries and even the prevention of wrinkles.

While not yet well known in the United States, grape seed extract is listed in pharmaceutical catalogues and prescribed by physicians in a number of European countries. For example, grape seed extract (sometimes shortened to GSE) has long been used for the prevention and treatment of a number of health problems related to the arteries and veins, including cardiovascular disease, varicose veins, and water retention, as well as damage to collagen, a factor in arthritis and even the condition of the skin. In the United States, grape seed extract is considered to be a food supplement or concentrate and is sold in drugstores and health-food stores.

Q. How was grape seed extract discovered?

A. It all started with red wine. Red wine has traditionally been considered to possess health-promoting benefits. But scientific confirmation of this, and discovery of the reason why it is so, are rather recent.

In 1933, the French researcher F. Dougnac found that more people in the wine-producing Mèdoc district lived well into old age as compared with people in other areas of the country. In the late 1940s and early 1950s Jack Masquelier, PhD, isolated compounds we now know as OPCs in the laboratory and demonstrated that red wine contained these compounds. From that point, it was an easy step to find that these beneficial compounds were concentrated in the seeds of the grapes from which the wine was made. An enormous amount of work was also performed in Germany on these compounds and again showed their health-promoting properties.

Then, in the late 1970s and early 1980s, scientists began noticing what they called the French Paradox. At about that time, the media had started reporting, and Americans had started becoming aware of, the dangers of fat and cholesterol. Yet, some scientists pointed out that the French people, as a group, ate all the foods they weren't "supposed to"—butter, cream, eggs, cheese, rich sauces, and so on—yet had less than half the incidence of heart disease as compared with people in the United

States. This sent health researchers scrambling to find other dietary factors that could explain this difference.

One obvious difference was the French love for wine, especially red wine. In the United States, wine tends to be something reserved for special occasions. In France it is a staple of the table. Initial studies seemed to back up the observation that the regular consumption of wine somehow had a preventive effect against many diseases. So researchers began to analyze the wine, looking for the source of its benefits. Again, their work took them to the grape seeds, or, more specifically, the skins of the grape seeds. Our current knowledge of grape seed extract emerged from research conducted at French medical centers, notably at the University of Bordeaux.

Q. Is grape seed extract one of the traditional plant-derived healers we have been hearing so much about in recent years?

A. Not in the form in which we now know it—grape seed extract as such has been in use only since the 1950s—but the active ingredients it contains have a very long history as part of healing traditions. For instance, some of the compounds it contains are also present in the berries, leaves, and flowering tops of the hawthorn plant, which has been used in Europe for centuries to treat heart and blood-vessel disorders, high blood pressure, and related conditions.

One of the most famous Asian longevity tonics is *he shou wu*. This herb also has been found to contain some of the same compounds as grape seed extract. The Chinese commonly use this root to treat high cholesterol, backache, and high blood pressure. Other healing plants that contain compounds similar to those in grape seed extract are the Japanese persimmon, various species of cinnamon, cranberries, members of the blueberry family, eucalyptus, many members of the rose family of plants, and tea. The outer coating of barley, considered by some to be the most health-promoting of all the grains, is another source. So while grape seed extract is a relatively recent entry in the field, the active ingredients it contains are present in many plants important to healing traditions around the world.

Q. How can a single supplement help so many different problems?

A. The conditions named above may seem very different because they affect different systems of the body, but, as we will see in later chapters, they have many important things in common. Also, grape seed extract contains a number of active phytochemicals (plant chemicals) that can exert effects throughout the body. The active phytochemicals in grape seed extract fall into a large group of compounds known as flavonoids.

Q. What are flavonoids?

A. Flavonoids are the primary pigments responsible for the many shades of pink, orange, red, violet, blue, and yellow colors in flowers and food. Anthocyanidins, one group of flavonoids, are pigments responsible for flower color and the coloration of fruits and other foodstuffs. They yield mostly red, violet, blue, and purple hues. Yellow flavonols, another group of flavonoids, produce yellow and orange colors.

As we will see, however, color is not the only, or even necessarily the most important, property of flavonoids. In fact, there are many flavonoids that are colorless but still have benefits. All in all, we have identified more than 4,000 chemically unique flavonoids in various plants and plant products, and it is a fairly sure bet we have only just scratched the surface when it comes to these compounds. Different flavonoids have been shown to possess antioxidant, anti-inflammatory, anti-allergenic, antiviral, anticarcinogenic, antimicrobial, antiparasitic, liver-protective, hypotensive (blood-pressure-lowering), antithrombotic (clot-preventing), and antihormonal properties.

Because they have so many beneficial effects, in some parts of the worlds, flavonoids are referred to as "vitamin P." In the United States, they are not generally considered vitamins.

Q. How can something be a vitamin in one country but not in another?

A. In order to be considered a vitamin in the United States, a substance must meet certain very specific criteria. One of these is that scientists must prove that a lack of sufficient quantities of the substance predictably results in a clearly identifiable deficiency syndrome. This is difficult to demonstrate with flavonoids because there are so many different flavonoids and they are naturally present in so many different foods. It would be a monumental task to create a truly flavonoid-free diet on any large scale, but this is what you would have to do in order to demonstrate the effects of a lack of flavonoids.

This situation is further complicated by the fact that flavonoids apparently have close interrelationships with other nutrients, particularly vitamin C. Vitamin C and the flavonoids are almost always found together in nature. Since we have long known about the effects of vitamin C, the common tendency is to attribute all the beneficial effects of fruits and other foodstuffs to the presence of that vitamin, even though there are flavonoids present as well. Nevertheless, some American authorities do call flavonoids "semi-essential nutrients."

Q. If flavonoids are found in so many foods, what makes grape seed extract special?

A. Grape seed extract contains three primary types of active flavonoids, classified according to their chemical structures. First, there are the monomers (which means "single units"). These are the catechins and epicatechins. Catechins have been shown to be effective in reducing the viability of many viruses, including the flu virus, the herpes simplex virus (the virus that causes cold sores and genital herpes), and even the virus responsible for some forms of chronic hepatitis. The antioxidant effects of the catechins offer protection against the formation of carcinogenic compounds known as nitrosamines during digestion, and thus help protect against stomach cancer. Furthermore, catechins may have protective effects against the development of atherosclerosis, the weakening of capillaries, and the buildup of excessive cholesterol and triglycerides (blood fats). Finally, catechin acts as a mild anti-inflammatory and antihistamine.

In addition to the monomers, there are the oligomers ("several units"). These, too, are good antioxidants and free-radical scavengers, but they do other things, as well, such as moderately lowering elevated blood pressure in some individuals. Lastly, there are the polymers ("many units"). The polymers may play a role in protecting against cancer in the intestinal tract. Studies suggest that a mixture of all these types of compounds, such as that naturally present in grape seed extract, may be more stable and beneficial than any of these substances alone.

On product labels, the active compounds in grape seed extract may be called PCO (which stands for procyanidolic oligomers) or, sometimes, OPC (for oligomères procyanodoliques, the equivalent in French).

Q. Why would I need to take supplements? Wouldn't I get enough flavonoids in the foods I eat?

A. Not if you eat the typical American diet. The Committee on Dietary Guidelines Implementation of the National Academy of Sciences has urged the adoption of dietary guidelines emphasizing the consumption of fruits and vegetables. We have had several years of the "Five a Day for Better Health" campaign, which urges that everyone eat five servings of fruits and vegetables every day. Yet only 23 percent of American adults eat the recommended number of servings of fruits and vegetables, and only 8 percent believe that they need to eat this number!

Q. What if I eat a vegetarian diet?

A. Often what we call a vegetarian diet is really just a meatless diet. And like most Americans, vegetarians may make the mistake of believing, for example, that a glass of fruit juice has the same value as the fruit itself. Unfortunately, eating a diet that relies upon carbohydrates as its main energy source does not guarantee that the diet is healthful. Moreover, not all carotenoids, flavonoids, and other plant compounds are created equal in their beneficial effect on the human body. The proanthocyanidins found in grape seed extract are especially active phytonutrients, and can be taken to provide nutritional "insurance" if you suspect that even your vegetarian diet is not all that it should be.

Q. How extensive is the research into the benefits of grape seed extract today?

A. It's very extensive. Remember that grape seed extract has been used pharmaceutically in Europe for decades. In fact, a number of European countries pay for prescriptions of grape seed extract through national health insurance plans. As this implies, grape seed extract had to undergo massive testing for a variety of conditions in order to qualify for this treatment.

Q. Are there other sources of the active compounds found in grape seed extract?

A. Yes, there are. Aside from red wine, good quality dark grape juice can contain significant amounts of the compounds found in grape seed extract. Unfortunately, grape juice also contains sugar, and therefore is not suitable for people who have diabetes or who want to control their intake of calories. The outside layers of barley are another source of proanthocyanidins, but this grain is not a common foodstuff for Americans. Similarly, some varieties of Japanese persimmon and the Chinese herb ho shu wu are good sources of these nutrients. OPCs are also found in the skins, seeds, barks, twigs, leaves, and blossoms of a number of other plants—but we do not usually eat these parts of plants. Grape seed extract therefore has the advantage of being easy to use and guaranteeing that you will get the amount of active compounds you want.

Q. Interest in plant-based supplements seems to be growing. Why?

A. The current revival of interest in traditional medicine, coupled with rapid advances in understanding the actions of a tremendous number of comounds found naturally in various plants, have led to a greater appreciation of phytonutrients in the past two or three decades.

Q. What exactly are phytonutrients?

A. *Phyto* simply means "plant" or "from plants." Most of our nutrients can be derived from plants. However, in current usage, the term *phytonutrients* is used to describe compounds other than the usual vitamins and minerals. There are many different categories classified as phytonutrients, among them, the carotenoids, catechins, flavonoids, genistein, indoles, isothiocyanates, phenolic acids, plant sterols, and so on. Most of these can turn on protective enzyme systems within our bodies, and some inhibit the production of cholesterol, impede the growth of hormone-sensitive cancers, and provide other benefits. Until recently, however, we were simply incapable of demonstrating scientifically the very wide range of benefits offered by various plant-derived antioxidants and free-radical scavengers. Even research into the antioxidant properties of long-known nutrients such as vitamin C and vitamin E is relatively recent. Previously, science tended to be interested only in obvious deficiency syndromes, such as scurvy. We now know that nutrition is often a much more subtle science, and many phytonutrients have far-reaching health benefits.

Q. How do I know if grape seed extract might help me?

A. Some people probably do stand to benefit more than would others from taking grape seed extract. For instance, as we will see in Chapters 3 and 4, it is especially useful for people with varicose veins, heart disease, edema, and other conditions related to the health of the blood vessels. Similarly, athletes, people with arthritis, and anyone subject to joint and cartilage injuries, bruising, and related problems may benefit from taking grape seed extract. One of the more interesting uses of grape seed extract is in preparation for surgery.

Even if you don't have any particular health problems, however, you can still benefit. Grape seed extract's antioxidant action can exert a long-term protective effect against the effects of aging and many degenerative diseases.

2.

The Super Antioxidant

Some of grape seed extract's most important benefits are due to its capability as an antioxidant. Antioxidants are substances that protect the body against harmful effects of free radicals. In recent years, scientists have been focusing a great deal of attention on free radicals and their possible role in aging and in many disorders whose causes have long been something of a mystery. In this chapter, we will look at free radicals and how they can harm the body, as well as what grape seed extract can do to protect against this damage.

Q. What are antioxidants?

A. In the simplest terms, antioxidants are substances that prevent a type of chemical reaction called *oxidation*. To truly understand what oxidation is, we have to look at free radicals. Free radicals are atoms and molecules that have a negative electric charge as a result of having one or more unpaired (unbalanced) electrons. Within an atom, there is a central nucleus containing protons, which are positively charged, and electrons that orbit around the nucleus, much as planets orbit around the sun. It is the nature of this type of structure to be more stable when the electrons are in pairs. If an atom or molecule contains an unpaired electron, it will seek to regain stability by either contributing the spare electron to or taking an electron from another molecule or atom. If it loses an electron, it is said to *be oxidized*; if it gains one, it is said to be *reduced*. Oxygen, which is present everywhere in the air, is the most common and active oxidizing agent, and has given its name to this process, although other compounds also can act as oxidizers. Many oxidation reactions result in some type of damage or decay. When iron undergoes oxidation, for example, the result is rust.

Q. Is oxidation always a bad thing?

A. No. In fact, some oxidation reactions are necessary for life. For example, our blood is capable of carrying oxygen to the cells thanks to an oxidation reaction that attaches oxygen to hemoglobin. Slow oxidation also provides the body with energy as we "burn" food in our cells. However, although oxidation is a necessary part of life, too much of it contributes to the aging process and disease. This is why is it often compared to the effect of oxidation on iron and referred to as the "rusting" of the body.

The problem for the body, therefore, is to control oxidation so that it takes place only where and when it is to our advantage. Otherwise, oxidation damages our tissues. Remember that free radicals are very unstable and tend to rob surrounding molecules of electrons in order to replace their missing ones. If they steal electrons from necessary molecules in the body's cells, the result is damage to the cells and, therefore, damage to the tissues of which those cells are a part. Worse, free radicals tend to activate chain reactions in which a series of thefts and donations of electrons takes place. In this process, stable compounds are robbed of electrons, become unstable, steal electrons in turn, and so forth. Free radicals interact with other substances and generate even more free radicals. Oxygen, for instance, is commonly turned into various free radicals. These are called oxygen-free radicals or reactive oxygen species.

Q. How exactly do antioxidants help?

A. Most antioxidants are compounds that donate electrons freely and therefore prevent harmful kinds of oxidation, such as oxidation of tissues, by substituting themselves. Vitamin C is a good example of an antioxidant that helps prevent the oxidation of proteins and fats in the body because it is oxidized in their place. Other antioxidants work by trapping certain metals, such as copper and iron, which can act to promote oxidation in the tissues. These two are the most common antioxidant mechanisms. Another action of many antioxidants is to act as a reducing agent. For instance, vitamin C is used in the body to reduce (or regenerate) oxidized vitamin E.

Q. Is there a difference between antioxidants and free-radical scavengers?

A. Technically, yes. While an antioxidant is a substance that steps in to intercept free radicals and prevent them from damaging tissues, a compound that terminates free-radical chain reactions is called a free-radical scavenger or a free-radical-chain breaker because it stops the formation of new free radicals.

Vitamin E and beta-carotene are such radical-chain breakers. However, the terms *antioxidant* and *free-radical scavenger* are often used interchangeably.

Q. Where do all these free radicals come from?

A. Free radicals have many sources. External sources include radiation and environmental toxins, such as smog and cigarette smoke. Internal sources can be divided into two groups. Some free radicals are normal byproducts of the metabolism of carbohydrates and other components of the diet. Others are normal byproducts of the workings of the immune system.

For example, the normal metabolism (breaking down) of sugars to provide energy, a process called glycolysis, creates free radicals. In glycolysis, glucose is broken down to yield lactic acid, and in the process releases energy. Because of the chemical nature of this process, which involves both bringing oxygen from the air into the body and appropriating hydrogen oxygen atoms from certain food-derived substances within the body, it readily creates types of free radicals known as superoxides and unstable peroxides.

The other prominent internal source of free radicals is the activity of the immune system. White blood cells called macrophages and neutrophils help defend against bacterial infections. When bacteria attack, these cells travel to the site of the infection and destroy the invaders by the release of what is termed an "oxygen burst." In this process, superoxide radicals, which are then converted into hydrogen peroxide, and hydroxyl radicals, are generated by the body to kill the bacterial cells. The immune cells therefore must have their own protection against the free radicals they generate, and they do. This protection comes from protective antioxidant enzymes and other substances that act as antioxidants.

Q. How exactly do free radicals affect health?

A. No matter what their source, free radicals can attack the membranes of cells, proteins, and fats in the bloodstream, the collagen that underlies the skin, and many other tissues. Free-radical damage is associated with aging and most if not all degenerative diseases.

The damage done by free radicals can show up in many ways. For instance, if free radicals damage a cell's strands of DNA—the cell's genetic blueprint—the cell can start to grow in abnormal ways, ultimately leading to cancer.

Q. Does that mean that grape seed extract might help prevent cancer?

A. Possibly. Antioxidants and free-radical scavengers in general can afford important protection against tumor promotion. Beyond this, OPCs such as those found in grape seed extract have been shown to effectively inhibit the effects of a known animal tumor promoter, a compound called phorbol ester. Similarly, extracts from the seeds of Japanese koshu wine grapes have been shown to inhibit the proliferation of cultured tumor cells, possibly by inhibiting enzymes necessary for cancer-cell growth. In many studies using animal models, catechin derivatives like those found in grape seed extract have been shown to be outstanding tumor inhibitors. Remarkably, grape seed extract seems to enhance the viability of normal cells while proving toxic to breast, lung, and other cancer cells.

Q. How do we get antioxidants?

A. Many antioxidants are supplied through the diet, and most of these come from fruits and vegetables. Some antioxidants are produced by the body, but certain specific nutrients—also found in fruits and vegetables—are needed for this to happen.

A number of vitamins, including vitamins A, C, and E, have antioxidant functions. The tocotrienols, nonvitamin compounds that are very close in structure to vitamin E, offer similar antioxidant protection. The B vitamins, while not necessarily antioxidants themselves, are nevertheless important cofactors in a number of the body's antioxidant actions. The vitaminlike compounds coenzyme Q_{10} and alpha-lipoic acid are particularly powerful antioxidants. There are also minerals that act as antioxidants, among them magnesium, which acts as a general antioxidant; selenium, which works together with vitamin E; and zinc, which is a component of superoxide dismutase (SOD), a powerful antioxidant enzyme produced by the body. Manganese also is important for production of SOD.

Q. Does that mean I can get all the antioxidants I need in a multivitamin pill?

A. Definitely not. While many vitamins and minerals are antioxidants, many more antioxidants are compounds found in whole foods. Carotenoids, for example, are a group of phytochemicals that have antioxidant benefits. Bright-yellow and orange fruits and vegetables, such as carrots and sweet potatoes, as well as deep-green vegetables, such as parsley and kale, are good sources of these nutrients. The best known of the carotenoids is beta-carotene, but there are many others, including lycopene, an especially powerful antioxidant found also in tomatoes and red grapefruit.

Catechins, which were mentioned in Chapter 1 as one of the beneficial components of grape seed extract, are also found in green tea and many berries. Flavonoids, also discussed in Chapter 1, are another group of antioxidants found in brightly colored fruits and vegetables. Other natural antioxidants that can be obtained through the diet include indoles, found in all members of the cabbage family; isothiocyanates, found in mustard, horseradish and radishes; and ellagic acid, found in abundance in strawberries.

Antioxidants can also be found in other, less well known, sources. Soybeans, for instance, contain substances called isoflavones. Genistein is the best known of these. It is an antioxidant that also has a number of special anticancer properties. Genistein can be found in some members of the cabbage family as well.

One particularly interesting feature of antioxidants is that different antioxidants are active in different parts in the body. For example, lycopene protects the prostate, while ellagic acid helps to prevent the formation of the carcinogen called *nitrosamine* in the digestive system. Superoxide dismutase protects the mitochondria, the energy-producing factories of the cells (and therefore also the most active site of free-radical production in the cells). Vitamins C and E are excellent antioxidants overall, but they are not nearly as protective of the prostate as lycopene nor as protective of the health of the eyes as some of the other carotenoids. OPCs have a particular affinity for protecting the walls of the arteries.

Q. If antioxidants are found in so many foods, why would I need to take supplements?

A. The Committee on Dietary Guidelines Implementation of the National Academy of Sciences recommends that we eat a minimum of five servings of fruits and vegetables every day. Unfortunately, more than three out of four Americans don't. So it is safe to say that at least 75 percent of all Americans do not get enough antioxidants in the foods they eat. Also, long and/or improper storage of fruits and vegetables robs many of the antioxidants they contain of their potency. So even if you follow the National Academy of Science's dietary guidelines, you may not be getting as much of the various antioxidants as you think because of today's farming and storage practices.

This is where supplements like grape seed extract come in. The flavonoids in grape seed extract act as antioxidants on their own and also protect other antioxidants, especially vitamin C, and keep it active. The catechins, one of the types of flavonoids in grape seed extract, are recognized as being powerful antioxidants. Grape seed extract's proanthocyanidins (the component often called *OPCs* on product labels), are among the most useful antioxidants found in the entire plant kingdom.

Q. How do we know that grape seed extract is an antioxidant?

A. In laboratory tests, OPCs are such potent antioxidants that they sometimes are said to be between 20 and 50 times as powerful as the antioxidant vitamins. An especially interesting aspect of grape seed extract is its ability to act as a point of contact between the two main classes of antioxidants, the water- and fat-soluble antioxidants. The compounds in grape seed extract are water-soluble, but they are also at least partially soluble in fats. As such, the OPCs of grape seed extract may be able to improve the interaction of the water- and fat-soluble antioxidants, such as the interaction between vitamin C and vitamin E. We will look at the specific ways in which this might benefit health in the chapters that follow.

In addition, the continuing research into flavonoids and related compounds has identified a substance called gallic acid as an especially powerful antioxidant. As it happens, gallic acid can be found attached to the proanthocyanidins found in grape seed extract. In this form, the gallic acid is called a gallate ester. Tests have confirmed that gallate esters are excellent antioxidants and free-radical scavengers. For instance, a group of Spanish scientists showed that the one gallate ester, known technically as proanthocyanidin B2-3'-o-gallate, which is found in grape seed extract, may be the most powerful antioxidant yet identified amongst the known proanthocyanidins.

Q. If I want to take antioxidants in supplement form, can I take just one or do I need to take a whole antioxidant "defense force?"

A. Most experts believe that antioxidants work best when taken in combination. In experimental and clinical tests, such antioxidant "cocktails" have turned out to be more powerful and effective than any one antioxidant taken on its own. There are many reasons for this. First, antioxidants can be either water soluble or fat soluble. Vitamin C is probably the best known water-soluble antioxidant; vitamin E the best known fat-soluble antioxidant. The body needs both types because they benefit different types of tissues. These two types of antioxidants also interact with each other in important ways. For instance, vitamin C, which is water soluble and so is found mostly in the blood, regenerates oxidized vitamin E, which is fat soluble and is found in cell membranes. Two-time Nobel-prize laureate Linus Pauling, who did much to publicize the benefits of vitamin C, took 1,800 milligrams (18 grams) of vitamin C each day, and often made a point of its ability to regenerate vitamin E.

Q. If I already take antioxidants, why would I want to take grape seed extract, too?

A. There are several reasons for using grape seed

extract in addition to other antioxidants. First, mixtures of antioxidants tend to be more effective than single ingredients. This has been shown over and over again in laboratory tests, and it makes sense in terms of what we know of the actions of these compounds. Second, we need both water-soluble and fat-soluble antioxidants for broad-ranging protection. Grape seed extract happens to have a peculiar affinity for the capillaries and the arteries, but it also is a premier antioxidant "team player" in that it protects other antioxidants and also acts as an interface between the water-soluble and the fat-soluble antioxidants. Also, while grape seed extract is a superb antioxidant, it also has other benefits to offer that are not directly related to its antioxidant qualities. As a result, it offers a great combination of potential health benefits in a single package.

3.

Cardiovascular Protection

Cardiovascular disease is the number-one cause of death in the United States, and we rank very near the top in terms of deaths per capita from this malady worldwide. There are two primary causes of death from cardiovascular disease: heart attack and stroke. According to the American Heart Association, roughly one million American adults die every year from heart attacks. This means that approximately one half of all deaths of adults in this country are a result of heart disease. Almost one-half million Americans die each year from strokes, which makes this a major threat in its own right. Clearly, finding ways to reduce these statistics is a major health priority.

Q. What exactly is cardiovascular disease?

A. Cardiovascular disease is a general term for disorders that affect the heart and/or blood vessels. There are many different types of cardiovascular disease, but the most common forms can all be linked to blockage and other problems affecting various blood vessels.

A heart attack, for instance, occurs because one or more of the arteries that supply the heart have become blocked. This blockage can result from fatty, sometimes calcified, deposits on the interior walls of the arteries that grow large enough to cut off blood flow. Sometimes the artery itself is only partially blocked by fatty deposits, but a blood clot may lodge in the narrowed artery and block it completely. In either case, blood flow to a section of the heart muscle is interrupted. This deprives the heart tissue of oxygen and, if the situation continues long enough, causes damage or death of localized areas of heart tissue.

In the case of stroke, the brain is affected, but the situation is much the same. Blood flow to an area of the brain is reduced or even blocked entirely by the narrowing of a major vessel by plaque and/or a blood clot. There is another scenario that can lead to stroke—if a blood vessel leaks or ruptures, that too can interrupt blood flow and lead to damage in an area of the brain.

Q. What causes the blood vessels to become blocked?

A. Generally, arteries are blocked by bits of fats that once were circulating in the bloodstream and then were deposited on the arterial walls. Other elements, such as calcium and dead white blood cells, may become bound up in the deposits as well. These deposits are referred to as plaque. Plaque not only narrows the passageway through which the blood must flow, but also makes the arteries less flexible, which in turn leads to high blood pressure. This is often the first sign of cardiovascular disease, and it usually precedes both heart attack and stroke.

Q. What makes the plaque form?

A. This is a complex process, and it is not completely understood; but we know a fair amount about some important aspects of it. The fatty material in the plaques comes from lipids (fats) circulating in the blood. There are a number of different blood lipids that are important here. Probably most important is cholesterol, a substance produced by the liver that is essential for the production of certain hormones and for maintaining cell walls throughout the body.

To get to the cells that need it, cholesterol travels through the bloodstream by means of molecules called lipoproteins. There are two primary types of cholesterol-carrying lipoproteins in the blood: low-density lipoproteins, or LDLs, which transports cholesterol from the liver to the cells, and high-density lipoproteins, or HDLs, which pick up excess cholesterol throughout the body and bring it back to the liver for disposal. If all excess cholesterol is picked up by the HDL molecules, a proper balance is maintained. However, certain factors, including a diet high in cholesterol and saturated fats, can result in more cholesterol than the HDLs can dispose of. This excess cholesterol may then be deposited on the walls of the arteries, initiating the formation of plaque.

The sheer quantity of cholesterol in the blood is not the only factor, however. Much recent work on the causes of cardiovascular disease suggests that fats in the blood that undergo oxidation are much more likely to become embedded in the lining of the arteries, poison the immune cells that attempt to remove them, and lead to the production of plaques. Also, plaques appear to be more likely to form in places where there have been minute breaks or tears in the lining of the arterial wall. Free radicals can directly attack the tissues and create weak spots and actual tears. The arteries' fundamental strength and resistance to tearing and damage may be involved as well; the blood vessels are placed under pressure with each beat of the heart, so a lack of proper structural integrity can easily lead to tiny cracks and other stress injuries. The body then takes steps to repair itself by "patching" the damaged areas. The problem is that the areas that are patched then tend to collect more and more patching material over time. Another factor that may play a role here is inflammation in the blood vessels. The end result is hardening of the arteries, high blood pressure (which itself increases the chance of damage to the lining of the arteries), and, in too many cases, heart attack or stroke.

Q. What can grape seed extract do to help?

A. Actually, it can do several things. First, grape seed extract is a powerful antioxidant. As such, it helps to prevent the oxidation of LDLs that make them more likely to stick to the blood-vessel walls, and also helps to control free radicals that might damage blood-vessel linings. Research presented in 1990 by Dr. David White of the University of Nottingham in England showed that OPCs reduce the formation of oxidized LDL cholesterol and foam cells, which are dead and dying white blood cells that had attempted to clear oxidized LDL from the arteries and ended up becoming embedded in the plaque instead.

A second protective effect of grape seed extracts concerns blood-clot formation. The formation of clots in the blood vessels is an important factor in heart attack and stroke; a clot that becomes lodged in a partially blocked artery can shut off the blood flow completely, depriving the heart or brain of oxygen. Controlling excessive clotting tendencies is therefore very important, and grape seed extract has demonstrated anti-clotting properties.

Finally, grape seed extract makes the linings of the arteries more resistant to damage. These tissues contain elastin and collagen, two important structural proteins. The flavonoids in grape seed extract act to inhibit the actions of enzymes that break down collagen-based tissues (more about this in Chapter 4). They therefore work with vitamin C to make (and keep) the structures of the blood vessels stronger and more elastic. Interestingly, the oligomers in grape seed extract appear to be more effective at preventing the oxidation of cholesterol, while catechin and the polymers seem to be more effective in protecting the artery walls from the actions of destructive enzymes.

Q. Can grape seed extract help high blood pressure?

A. Yes. In addition to reducing the formation of plaque, which usually precedes the development of high blood pressure, grape seed extract OPCs have a mild inhibiting effect on angiotensin I-converting enzyme (ACE). This enzyme, which is produced in the kidneys, influences blood-fluid balances and contributes to high blood pressure. This effect of OPCs is similar to that of drugs known as ACE inhibitors, but grape seed extract works more slowly and much more safely than these drugs. For example, pregnant women should not take ACE-inhibitor drugs because of risks to the fetus. In contrast, grape seed extract is a safe constituent of food. Animal experiments have confirmed that grape seed extract can sometimes reduce elevated blood pressure by as much as 20 percent.

Q. How were all these benefits of grape seed extract for the heart discovered?

A. Most Americans are familiar with the idea that eating a diet high in fat and cholesterol is an important contributor to blood-vessel blockage. After all, if there is less fat circulating in your blood, it stands to reason that less will be deposited in the arteries. But it turns out that this is only part of the equation. This is where the so-called French paradox came in.

In the late 1970s, researchers noticed a very interesting phenomenon. They were looking at the mortality rates from heart attack in men aged fifty-five to sixty-four in countries around the world. In the United States and the Scandinavian countries, these rates were comparatively high; in France, Italy, and Switzerland, they were lower. Now, the French men in this study ate more saturated fat and cholesterol than the Americans did, and got a greater percentage of their total daily calories as fat. They also smoked much more, another risk factor for heart disease. Yet they had a heart-attack rate that was only about 40 percent that of their American counterparts.

When the researchers charted the rates of death from heart attack against total wine consumption, they found that there was a remarkable correlation between the two. Specifically, France had the highest average daily wine consumption, followed very closely by Italy, and then by Switzerland. And these three had the lowest heart-attack-death rates of all the countries surveyed.

Q. Does that really prove that the wine is what made the difference?

A. Not entirely; the whole answer is probably much more complex than that. There are other important differences in eating habits, too. For instance, the French and Italians eat far more fresh foods, especially fresh vegetables, than Americans do. Moreover, we tend to like our foods much sweeter than Europeans do, and this, too, makes a difference. So while a French person is more likely to eat a whole orange, with all of its fiber and vitamins and minerals, an American is more likely to drink the juice of the orange, which concentrates the sugars but loses virtually everything else of nutritional value. Thus, while the traditional French diet may be higher in fat, it is also much richer in vitamins, minerals, fiber other valuable plant compounds. The traditional French diet also has only 5.6 percent of the amount of sugar found in the American diet. In any case, it is obvious that fat alone is not the problem.

This is not to discount the importance of the wine, however. The Copenhagen Heart Study, whose results were published in the *British Medical*

Journal in 1995, reported that subjects who consumed three to five glasses of wine daily over the twelve-year course of the study had only half the mortality risk of those who did not drink at all. Beer and liquor did not confer the same protection, suggesting that something other than the alcohol in the wine—often thought of as the "active ingredient"—was responsible for this benefit.

Q. Does all wine provide the same protection?

A. No. Only red wine seems to have this benefit. The reason for this lies in the way wine is made in France, Italy, and the United States. Red wine is left in contact with the grape seeds, skins, and stems for two to three weeks, which is long enough for it to acquire significant amounts of antioxidants—proanthocyanidins (OPCs) and catechins from the seeds and anthocyanidins from the skins. A number of other components are involved as well. All in all, the process used in fermenting red wine makes for a mixture rich in antioxidant compounds. White wine, in contrast, is made from the juice that is pressed from the grapes, so it lacks all these beneficial substances. It is true that in some parts of Eastern Europe, white wines are left in contact with the grape seeds long enough to get significant amounts of proanthocyanidins, but this practice imparts an astringent taste not generally appreciated by Western palates.

Of course, grape seed extract allows you to gain the benefits of these antioxidants easily and conveniently, without worrying about such things as fermentation processes or alcohol.

Q. Have there been human studies showing the benefits of grape seed extract for cardiovascular disorders?

A. Yes. Grape seed extract is often prescribed in Europe for various circulatory conditions. In addition to cardiovascular problems, these include a sensation of heaviness in the legs, restless legs or night cramps, edema (fluid retention), and others. Numerous clinical trials have been written up in medical and scientific literature. Most have found statistically significant positive results with supplementation of 150 to 300 mg of grape seed extract per day. As a rule, it takes from one to three months for symptoms to improve. This is because grape seed extract does not so much treat symptoms as provide the body with the tools with which it can repair itself.

Animal experiments confirm grape seed extract's ability to reduce platelet aggregation—the tendency of the platelets in the blood to stick together and form clots. Serge Renaud, PhD, of the French National Institute of Health and Medical Research, performed an elaborate series of experiments in which he gave different groups of animal subjects access to various liquids to drink. The control group got plain water; other groups got white wine standardized to 6 percent alcohol; red wine standardized to 6 percent alcohol; water with 6-percent alcohol added; and water with 6-percent alcohol plus 0.03 percent grape seed extract. What he found was that all the alcoholic beverages at first reduced platelet aggregation by about 59 percent, but that within 18 hours after all alcohol had been withdrawn, the subjects experienced a "rebound" effect, in which platelet aggregation increased again. As compared with the control group, the water plus alcohol group had a 129-percent rebound and the white wine group had a 46-percent rebound. In contrast, the red wine group and the water plus alcohol plus grape seed extract showed the initial lowering effect with no rebound effect at all. This clearly demonstrated the ability of grape seed extract and red wine to protect against blood clots with no negative consequences afterward.

4.

From Allergies and Arthritis to Varicose Veins and Wrinkles

So far, we have seen how grape seed extract can protect your body from the assaults of free radicals and decrease the dangers of cardio-vascular disease. Though dramatic and important, these effects are not all that this versatile extract has to offer. In this chapter, we will look at the possible benefits of grape seed extract for people with allergies, arthritis, varicose veins, or hemorrhoids. You may be surprised to learn that it can even fight wrinkles and help your complexion.

Q. How can a single supplement benefit conditions as different as allergies, arthritis, and hemorrhoids—not to mention wrinkles?

A. Although these seem like very different conditions affecting entirely different parts and systems of the body, in fact they are related to one another in certain important ways. Specifically, all of them result, directly or indirectly, from the activity of immune system.

When the body perceives that it is under attack from dangerous outside invaders, such as bacteria, a type of cell called the *mast cell* responds by releasing a number of chemicals to fight back. These chemicals include histamine; hyaluronidase, an enzyme; serotonin, a neurotransmitter, and bradykinin, an amino-acid compound. These substances trigger and regulate the inflammatory response that results in localized redness, warmth, fluid retention, an increase in the permeability of small vessels, and other changes. While these changes can cause discomfort, they take place because they boost the body's infection-fighting capability. An increase in temperature, for instance, makes it more difficult for many microorganisms to survive. The redness is a sign that the blood supply to the area has been increased in an attempt to bring more infection-fighting white blood cells to the area, and the increased permeability of the capillaries makes it easier for the white blood cells to exit into the tissues where they are needed to fight the invaders.

Thus, an allergic reaction is essentially a case of the body responding to a normally harmless substance with all the weapons it usually employs to fight disease. The release of histamine causes itching, sniffling, sneezing, and possibly, an inflammatory reaction in the skin (hives) as the body tries to kill or expel something it has determined (however inappropriately) is a danger. Catechin, a component of grape seed extract, can help reduce the allergic response because it inhibits the action of histidine decarboxylase, an enzyme involved in the formation of histamine.

Q. How does that relate to the other problems you mentioned?

A. Arthritis, varicose veins, hemorrhoids, and, yes, even wrinkles, can all be traced to the activity of the immune system as well. Remember that the enzyme hyaluronidase is one of the substances released by the mast cells as part of the immune response. This enzyme has the effect of breaking down many tissue components that are built from the protein collagen. When triggered by histamine, hyaluronidase splits apart chains of molecules that undergird the structure of many of the body's tissues. Presumably, this is part of the mechanism by which the capillaries are made more permeable so that white blood cells can exit easily to fight infection. But it also can have the effect of damaging many collagen-based tissues, which can lead to a variety of problems and may even be implicated in metastasis, the migration of tumor cells from one part of the body to another.

Q. What is collagen, and why is it important?

A. Many of us have heard of collagen as an ingredient in skin creams. In fact, collagen is the most abundant protein in the body, and it is found in many different kinds of tissues. Collagen is constructed from chains of amino acids (the basic building blocks of all proteins), plus specialized sugars that influence its strength, that are woven together to form strands, or fibers. These fibers take various shapes to match the body's needs. Thin layers of collagen form the skin; similar layers line the veins and arteries. Ropelike collagen structures form the tendons. In addition to its basic constituents, the synthesis of collagen requires vitamin C and the minerals copper, iron, manganese, silicon, and zinc.

Q. What does collagen have to do with arthritis?

A. Arthritis is a general term for inflammation of the joints. It can cause pain and a limited range of movement. Osteoarthritis is a type of arthritis that comes about from wear and tear; rheumatoid arthritis is a type of this condition that appears to be an autoimmune disease—a disorder in which the immune system mistakenly begins to attack its own tissues.

Collagen is a factor in arthritis because, in two of its many shapes, this protein supplies the basic scaffolding of the bones and also forms cartilage. Within the joints, cartilage forms a rubbery layer that protects the ends of bones from rubbing against each other as the joint goes through its normal range of motion.

If you looked minutely at the structure of cartilage, you would see that it consists of collagen webbing filled with substances called proteoglycans. Collagen is also a preliminary building block for the proteoglycans, and like collagen, the proteoglycans are composed of amino acids and sugars. One important feature of these huge molecules is their affinity for water. When they are not under pressure, they draw water into themselves; when pressure is applied, they release some of this liquid. The result is a kind of cushioning effect within the joints; it allows the cartilage to be compressed as the joint changes shape with movement, while still preventing the bones from grinding against one another as the joint moves. In arthritis, the cartilage gradually breaks down and, without its cushioning effect, the bones rub and scrape against each other with every movement, resulting in inflammation, pain, and a limited range of motion.

Q. What causes the cartilage to break down?

A. As mentioned earlier, wear and tear can be a factor, but another factor, perhaps even more significant, is the effect of collagen- and proteoglycan-destroying enzymes such as hyaluronidase. These damaging enzymes are often produced within the joints themselves.

Q. Why would the body attack its own tissues with damaging enzymes?

A. The body is in a state of a dynamic balance between processes that build up and those that tear down. Worn out and damaged tissue is broken down and removed, and new tissue is generated to take its place. The tearing-down phase of renewal is most often performed by specific enzymes, such as elastase, collagenase, and hyaluronidase (the suffix *-ase* means "to split"; thus, *collagenase* means "to split collagen").

Chondrocytes are cells responsible for the repair and regeneration of cartilage tissue. This is a constant process and involves both the removal of worn-out cartilage and the synthesis of new cartilage. Enzymes produced by the chondrocytes tear down cartilage as proteoglycans synthesized by the chondrocytes renew it.

Both of these steps are necessary, and a balance needs to be maintained for joint health. However, the process by which old cartilage is destroyed is accelerated by inflammation and injury. Remember, the inflammatory response involves the production of hyaluronidase and related enzymes. This can result in cartilage being destroyed faster than the chondrocytes can replace it, and the end result of that is arthritis. Many sports injuries can produce similar results.

Q. How can grape seed extract help?

A. Grape seed extract acts both to reduce the free-radical formation associated with inflammation and to inhibit overly aggressive enzymatic destruction of collagen-based tissues. Both of these are important factors in arthritis. In fact, a number of specialty antiarthritis products are now incorporating grape seed extract into formulas designed to promote joint repair.

Studies have shown that compounds in grape seed extract reduce the release of histamine and the activation of hyaluronidase. For example, research in Japan found that both gallic acid and OPCs inhibit the activation of hyaluronidase. Other research has shown that catechin inhibits the activation of hyaluronidase. OPCs also appear to be potent inhibitors of elastases.

Incidentally, this is the same mechanism involved in grape seed extract's effect on blood vessels. Increases in collagen- and elastin-degrading enzymes result in the weakening of artery walls. By stabilizing collagen and elastin, compounds in grape seed extract may help to prevent tiny cracks in the arteries that lead to the deposition of plaque in the vessel walls.

Q. How can varicose veins benefit from grape seed extract?

A. A varicose vein is a vein that has become stretched and swollen. As a result, the one-way valves that normally work to force the blood back to the heart can no longer close properly in the enlarged areas, and the blood pools there, stretching the vein further. Veins in the leg are most likely to develop this problem, but it can occur anywhere in the body.

The underlying cause of varicose veins is weakness of the walls of the veins. The walls of varicose veins differ from those of normal veins in that they have lost much of their collagen content and have a higher than normal level of proteoglycans, particularly hyaluronic acid. This change, which results in a loss of tissue strength, has been explained as a result of the activity of protein-degrading (collagen-destroying) enzymes, such as hyaluronidase, and of free-radical damage. Grape seed extract offers two benefits here. First, as we saw in Chapter 2, it contains flavonoids that are powerful antioxidants. Second, it can decrease the enzyme attacks that weaken and destroy collagen.

The stabilizing effects of compounds in grape seed extract on collagen have been known for a long time. Researchers reported years ago that collagen treated with derivatives of catechin, both in the test tube and in animal studies, showed increased stability.

Q. Have there been any studies on people that show grape seed extract to be helpful for varicose veins?

A. Yes. In fact, quite a number of clinical trials have been performed in France showing that OPCs have positive effects with respect to capillary fragility and varicose veins. These trials typically used grape seed extracts as the source of OPCs. There have also been good results with sports injuries and fluid retention following surgery. In most of these trials, subjects received 150 to 300 mg of OPCs a day in divided doses.

Q. What about hemorrhoids?

A. Many people don't know this, but a hemorrhoid is actually a type of varicose vein. The main thing that distinguishes hemorrhoids is their uncomfortable location. So what's true for varicose veins should also be true for hemorrhoids.

Q. Let's talk about wrinkles now. Are they related to collagen damage also?

A. Yes, but that's not the whole story. The skin is largely made up of collagen and a similar protein, elastin. Grape seed extract protects the skin by reducing damage to these proteins from overly aggressive enzyme action. But the flavonoids in grape seed extract also help the skin by protecting vitamin C. One of the important functions of vitamin C in the body happens to be in the synthesis of new collagen and elastin. Grape seed extract, therefore, works on both sides of the equation here—both slowing down the destruction and promoting the production of these vital proteins.

In addition, grape seed extract, as a powerful free-radical scavenger and antioxidant, helps to protect against the damage done by exposure to radiation from the sun and environmental toxins, such as harmful chemicals, and by smog. One sign of damage due to the sun's ultraviolet rays is *erythema*, a reddening of the skin due to congestion of capillaries underlying the skin. Tests with human subjects have shown that OPCs can reduce the occurrence of erythema brought on by exposure to the sun. The positive effects of grape seed extract are so broad that some experts in the field have called the OPCs found in grape seed extract a "skin cosmetic in a capsule."

5.

Relief From PMS and Other Benefits

As we have seen, grape seed extract is especially beneficial in two areas—antioxidant protection and protection of collagen. Antioxidants, of course, are important for maintaining the proper functioning of metabolism and the immune system, and even communication amongst cells. Collagen-based tissues are so fundamental to human physiology that they might even be called the skeleton's skeleton. It should, therefore, come as no surprise that grape seed extract can be useful for almost any condition that involves the health of the blood vessels and the actions of free radicals.

In this chapter, we will turn our attention to the ways in which this supplement can benefit a number of other health problems. These conditions include premenstrual syndrome, digestive-tract ulcers, and age-related problems, such as declining eyesight and brain function.

Q. What is premenstrual syndrome, and what causes it?

A. Premenstrual syndrome (probably better known by the abbreviation PMS) is a broad term for a group of symptoms many women experience during their monthly hormonal fluctuations. Medical researchers have now broken the general category of PMS down into a number of subcategories, but most PMS sufferers go through cyclic hormonal imbalances—specifically, periods when levels of the sex hormone estrogen are too high and those of progesterone, which acts to balance the effects of estrogen, are too low. This monthly imbalance gives rise to a wide variety of symptoms, including anxiety, nervousness, and mood swings. Other problems associated with PMS include food cravings and fatigue. These are associated with imbalances in hormonelike substances called prostaglandins and problems in the regulation of blood-sugar levels. Another primary set of PMS-related symptoms includes breast tenderness and fluid retention.

Q. Can grape seed extract help in a condition with causes and symptoms as complicated as those of in PMS?

A. The results speak for themselves. In one study, 165 women with one or more physical complaints during the second half of their monthly cycles took 200 mg of grape seed extract per day from the fourteenth through the twenty-eighth days of the cycle. Within two months, 60 percent of the women found that their physical disorders had disappeared; within four months, 80 percent found that they were free of symptoms. As a further benefit, 66 percent of the women who had also suffered from dysmenorrhea (painful menstruation) were free of those symptoms as well by the end of four months. The reason for these benefits is not entirely certain, but it seems likely that antioxidant actions of grape seed extract are a significant factor, since similar improvements have been noted among women taking vitamin E, another antioxidant.

Q. What can grape seed extract do for ulcers?

A. Scientists have known for many years that stress is an important factor in the development of stomach and upper gastrointestinal tract ulcers. Recently, much has been made of the role of a strain of bacteria in stomach ulcers. While bacteria may indeed be important, studies have demonstrated time and again that high levels of stress will reliably lead to the development of stomach ulcers.

How? Many experts believe that ulcers are caused by damage to the stomach wall that results from the stress-induced release of excessive amounts of histamine in the stomach. As we saw in Chapter 4, histamine is an active component of the inflammatory response. OPCs such as those found in grape seed extract act to reduce the body's release of histamine.

Some ulcers are not so much tied to stress, but result from injury to the stomach lining by nonsteroidal anti-inflammatory drugs (NSAIDs), such as aspirin, ibuprofen, and similar agents. The types of flavonoids found in grape seed extract have been reported to provide significant protection against this type of injury. Grape seed extract may, therefore, be useful in controlling at least two common causes of gastric ulcers.

Q. Many of us are worried about keeping our brains functioning optimally as we get older. Can grape seed extract help with brain function?

A. Actually, older people are not the only ones who may benefit mentally from taking grape seed extract—younger people can, too. As we have seen, OPCs reduce the fragility of the capillaries, including those in the brain. This helps to ensure a good supply of oxygen and nutrients to the brain, which is of increasing importance as we age. Moreover, grape seed extract may help to improve circulation in general, which is another key element to maintaining peak brain function. Finally, although we don't normally think of the brain as requiring much energy, in fact it is an important consumer of glucose and oxygen. This means that it is subject to the production of free radicals arising from normal metabolism. Grape seed extract's antioxidant properties can help protect the brain from damage due to free radicals. If you don't always eat five servings of fruits and vegetables daily, grape seed extract can provide some of the nutrients you're missing.

Q. Vision is another function that often declines with age. Can grape seed extract help to protect the eyes?

A. Yes. Studies have shown that OPCs can benefit sight in two main ways. Under normal circumstances, the eye adapts from bright to dim light through the activation of a pigment in the retina called *rhodopsin*, or visual purple, that is made from protein and a form of vitamin A. As it does with vitamin C, grape seed extract appears to enhance some of the functions of vitamin A. In one study, 98 of 100 test subjects given 200 mg of OPCs daily experienced an improvement in their ability to adapt to low light levels after being exposed to bright light. Their resistance to "blinding" from the sudden exposure to bright light similarly improved. This test result suggests that OPCs may help us to maintain night vision as we age.

Another exciting finding regarding grape seed extract and vision concerns diabetic retinopathy. In this condition, which is associated with insulin-dependent diabetes, eyesight is gradually damaged due to multiple problems within the eye, including microaneurisms (weak areas in veins that "balloon" into surrounding tissues and may burst), hemorrhages (bleeding), swelling of the macula (a small spot on the retina responsible for fine central vision), waxy exudations, the development of proliferative lesions (spreading areas of fibrous tissue), inflammation, and tissue degeneration. Several studies using dosages of 100 to 200 mg OPCs daily have been successful in reducing the damage that is characteristic of diabetic retinopathy. Microaneurisms, hemorrhages, swelling, inflammation, waxy exudate, inflammation, and proliferative lesions all responded positively to OPCs. Typically, 60 to 80 percent of the subjects in these studies experienced an improvement within one to three months, depending on the dosage and the severity of the condition.

Q. Are there other possible benefits from grape seed extract?

A. Two areas we have not considered up to this point, but that show real promise, are topical use (that is, applying grape seed extract directly to the skin) and dental applications. Some research has found that applying grape seed extract to the skin in cream or lotion form can protect the skin against free-radical damage associated with exposure to the sun and environmental pollutants. In the dental arena, the astringent properties of red wine have long been considered to protect the teeth and the gums against attack by bacteria. Because vitamin-C deficiency affects the tissues of the mouth, and grape seed extract increases the activity of vitamin C, it seems logical that grape seed extract would benefit dental health. This is an area that deserves further research.

6.

How to Take Grape Seed Extract

Before taking any dietary supplement, you should know how much to take and how to take it. It is also wise to research its effects and safety record. In the preceding chapters, we have looked in detail at the many effects of this versatile extract. In this, the final chapter of *All About Grape Seed Extract*, we will look at exactly how to take it. We will also examine its safety.

Q. What is the recommended daily dose of grape seed extract?

A. Most people who take grape seed extract for health problems take 300 mg or more per day. As a preventive, a healthy person might consider taking 50 to 250 mg daily. If you are active and athletic, particularly if you engage in contact sports, you may want to keep your intake toward the higher end of this range.

When you first begin to take grape seed extract, it is a good idea to take a *loading dose* of 300 mg daily for up to three months, then cut back to a lower daily *maintenance dose*. The purpose of the loading dose is to fully saturate the tissues with OPCs. This may take anywhere from ten days to three months, depending upon your body and the severity of any condition you are trying to treat. In clinical studies, the usual loading dose is 1.5 mg per pound of body weight. This translates into 225 mg if you weigh about 150 pounds, 180 mg if you weigh about 120, and 270 mg if you weigh about 180. The appropriate maintenance dose is usually one-third the loading dose. However, if you have a very large frame or serious health concerns, you might want to take loading and maintenance doses that are higher than these. Children, depending upon body weight, should take one-half of the adult dosage.

In general, it is best not to take the entire daily dose at once, but to split it up into two or three equal parts and take them at intervals over the course of the day.

Q. How will I know if grape seed extract is working?

A. It depends on why you are taking it, of course. If you are using it for a specific health problem, you can judge by your symptoms. But there are various ways in which people benefit from supplements, and not all of these benefits are immediate. The rule of thumb is that the better your overall health, the less likely it is that you will notice an immediate difference with any supplement. Keep in mind, though, that grape seed extract may be most important for its ability to prevent or delay the onset of various health problems. As we have seen, grape seed extract is a powerful antioxidant—a substance that neutralizes hazardous free radicals *before* they can damage your body. Damage from free radicals can show up in many forms, including cancer, heart disease, and arthritis, but this kind of damage often takes many years to appear. So even if you are in excellent health and not seeking relief from any particular problems now, grape seed extract can exert a long-term protective effect. In this sense, grape seed extract is really a special "food" that can be used to maintain health, not just a supplement to take when something goes wrong. After all, it is always easier to prevent trouble than to correct damage.

Q. How safe is grape seed extract?

A. Grape seed extract has been used in Europe for therapeutic purposes for several decades. In fact, grape seed OPCs are prescribed by doctors and are listed in pharmaceutical catalogs. European doctors prescribe it to protect against damage to the cardio-vascular system and excessive capillary permeability, to improve resistance to trauma, and to reduce fluid retention and a feeling of heaviness in the legs. Side effects are rare. Jack Masquelier, PhD, probably the world's leading expert on OPCs, has said that grape seed extract is not only safe but even health-promoting in conditions such as pregnancy.

The reason that grape seed extract is so safe is that it really is a type of food. It is not a drug. Rather, it is a concentration of special health-enhancing flavonoids. A few individuals with very sensitive stomachs sometimes experience slight stomach upset after taking it, but this is easily remedied by reducing the dosage and by taking it with meals. There have been no known toxic effects over many years and with countless users of grape seed extract.

Q. Is there anyone who shouldn't take grape seed extract?

A. As a food supplement, grape seed extract is extraordinarily safe. Unless you are actually allergic to grapes—truly an uncommon allergy—it is unlikely that there would be any reason you shouldn't take grape seed extract. And considering all the benefits this supplement has to offer, there are many, many reasons to give it a try.

Conclusion

Throughout most of Europe, and especially in France, the moderate consumption of red wine is a cultural tradition. In recent years, it has been found to have definite health-promoting properties as well. Now the many benefits of this healthful tradition are available in a convenient, standardized form, as grape seed extract.

No one compound can prevent or treat all health problems, but decades of use in Europe have shown grape seed extract to be remarkably versatile. Modern research into the benefits of OPCs, the active ingredients in this extract, continues at a brisk pace, but we already have learned enough to cast considerable light on how grape seed extract works. Research shows that it is a powerful antioxidant and free-radical scavenger that works extremely well in conjunction with other antioxidants, such as vitamins A and C. Moreoever, grape seed extract has a special affinity for the collagen-based tissues of the body. These include the linings of the arteries and the veins, the cartilage of the joints, and the skin.

Finally, grape seed extract is a safe way to include a food-derived form of "health insurance" in your everyday life. It deserves a prominent place in any nutritional supplement program.

Glossary

Antioxidant. A substance that prevents or controls oxidation (*see* Oxidation). In the body, antioxidants protect tissues and cells from damage by free radicals. The vitamins C and E are examples of antioxidants.

Atherosclerosis. A disease in which fatty plaques develop on the interior walls of arteries and lead to progressive damage. If extensive, these plaques can narrow or even completely obstruct the arteries and cut off the flow of blood.

Atom. The smallest unit of an element such as hydrogen or iron. Atoms become linked to form molecules.

Catechin. A type of flavonoid classified as a monomer found in grape seed extract.

Cholesterol. A type of lipid produced by the liver that is essential for the production of certain hormones and for maintaining cell walls throughout the body. If present in excessive amounts, however, it can lead to atherosclerosis.

Cofactor. A substance that is necessary for the action or production of another compound. For example, vitamin C is a cofactor in the production of collagen.

Collagen. The body's main structural protein. Collagen is a primary building block for bone, cartilage, tendons, ligaments, skin, and other connective tissue.

DNA. Material found in the nucleus of each cell of the body that contains the genetic code that controls that cell. *DNA* stands for *deoxyribonucleic* acid.

Elastin. A protein related to collagen that is a primary component of elastic tissue fibers found in the skin, the lungs, and the walls of the arteries.

Electron. A component of an atom that carries a negative elecrical charge. The simplest atom, hydrogen, consists of one proton (a positive charge in the nucleus) and one electron in orbit around the proton.

Enzyme. A type of protein molecule that speeds up the rate of a particular biochemical reaction.

Epicatechin. A type of flavonoid classified as a monomer found in grape seed extract.

Flavonoid. Any of a class of active compounds found in plants. Some flavonoids are the elements that impart color to flowers and fruits. All have antioxidant properties.

Free radical. An atom or molecule that has an unpaired electron, making it highly unstable and likely to react with other substances. Because of this, free radicals can damage the body at the cellular level.

HDL. The type of molecule that transports cholesterol through the bloodstream and to the liver for disposal. Sometimes called "good cholesterol." *HDL* stands for *high-density lipoprotein*.

LDL. The type of molecule that transports cholesterol through the bloodstream to the cells for energy and hormone production. Sometimes called "bad cholesterol." *LDL* stands for *low-density lipoprotein*.

Lipid. Any of a group of substances including fats and oils, and compounds soluble in fats and oils. Lipids are a necessary component of all cell membranes and are used for both energy and hormone production.

Macula. A yellowish spot on the retina of the eye that is chiefly responsible for visual acuity in the center of the visual field.

Metabolic pathway. The steps or ordered pathway through which a particular biochemical process is accomplished. For instance, there is a metabolic pathway for the production of energy from carbohydrates.

Metabolism. (1) The totality of biochemical processes of the body. (2) The pathway and fate of a particular aspect of activity in the body, such as the metabolism of fats.

Mitochondria. Structures found within cells that use nutrients from food to produce energy. The mitochondria are the sites of much of the free-radical generation that occurs in the body, and consequently are likely to be the object of attack from free radicals.

Molecule. The smallest unit of a substance that retains the properties of that substance. Molecules are composed of one or more atoms.

Monomer. Chemically, a single unit. Monomers can be linked together to form chains. A chain of monomers is a polymer.

Oligomer. Chemically, a polymer consisting of two, three, or, in some cases, four monomers linked together (these are called a dimer, a trimer, and a tetramer, respectively).

OPC. A type of flavonoid classified as an oligomer found in grape seed extract. *OPC* stands for *oligomères procyanodoliques*, which is French for "procyanidolic oligomers."

Oxidation. A chemical reaction in which an electron, the unit of negative electrical charge, is taken from an atom to balance an unpaired electron in another atom or molecule. Oxidation reactions usually are associated with some type of spoilage or decay. An example is the rusting of iron.

PCO. Procyanidolic oligomers (*see* OPC).

Polymer. Chemically, any chain of monomers. Usually used of polymers containing more than four units (those consisting of two, three, or four units are usually called oligomers).

Proanthocyanidin. Any of a number of flavonoids constructed from catechin and/or epicatechin that yield the red color of anthocyanidins when treated chemically in a specific fashion. The oligomers and the polymers in grape seed extract are proanthocyanidins. The term is commonly used interchangably with *procyanidin*.

References

Baumann J, Wurm G, and von Bruchhausen F, "Hemmung der Prostaglandinsynthetase durch Flavonoide und Phenolderivate im Vergleich mit deren $O^{2-\bullet}$-Radikalfängereigenshaften," *Archiv der Pharmazie* 313 (1980): 330–337.

Clemetson CAB and Andersen L, "Plant polyphenols as antioxidants for ascorbic acid," *Annals of the New York Academy of Sciences* 136 (1966): 339–378.

Da Silva JMR et al., "Radical scavenging capacity of different procyanidins from grape seeds," *Royal Society of Chemistry* (January 1990): 79–80

Da Silva JMR et al., "Procyanidin dimers and trimers from grape seeds," *Phytochemistry* 30 (4) (1991): 1259–1264.

Das N and Ratty A, "Effects of Flavonoids on Induced Non-Enzymatic Lipid Peroxidation," in *Plant Flavonoids in Biology and Medicine*, Vol. 1 (New York: Alan R. Liss, Inc., 1986): 243–247.

Demrow HS, Slane PR, and Folts JD, "Administration of wine and grape juice inhibits in vivo platelet activity and thrombosis in stenosed canine coronary arteries," *Circulation* 91 (1995): 1182–1188.

Doutremepuich JD, Barbier A, and Lacheretz F, "Effect of endotelon (procyanidolic oligomers) on experimental acute lymphedema of the rat hind-limb," *Lymphology* 24 (1991): 135–139.

Feine-Haake G, "A new therapy for venous diseases with 3,3′,4,4′,5,7- ," *Zeitschrift für Allgemeinmedizin* (30 June 1975).

Fuhrman B, Lavy A, and Aviram M, "Consumption of red wine with meals reduces the susceptibility of human plasma and low-density lipoprotein to lipid peroxidation," *The American Journal of Clinical Nutriton* 61 (3) (1995): 549–554.

Gali HU et al., "Comparison of the inhibitory effects of monomeric, dimeric, and trimeric procyanidins on the biochemical markers of skin tumor promotion in mouse epidermis in vivo," *Planta Medica* 60 (1994): 235–239.

Gendre PMJ, Laparra J, and Barraud E, "Effet protecteur des oligomères procyanidoliques sur le lathyrism expérimental chez la rat," *Annales Pharmaceutiques Françaises* 3 (1) (1985) 61-71.

Glories Y, "Anthocyanins and tannins from wine: organoleptic properties," in *Plant Flavonoids in Biology and Medicine*, Vol. 2 (New York: Alan R. Liss, Inc., 1988): 123–134.

Grønbæk M et al., "Mortality associated with moderate intakes of wine, beer, or spirits," *British Medical Journal* 310 (1995): 1165–1169.

Harborne JB, ed., *The Flavonoids* (New York: Chapman and Hall, 1988): 1–62.

Haslam E, *Plant Polyphenols: Vegetable Tannins Revisited* (Cambridge, England: Cambridge University Press, 1989).

Kühnau J, "The flavonoids. A class of semi-essential food components: their role in human nutrition," *World Review of Nutrition and Dietics* 24 (1976) 117–191.

Masquelier J, et al., "Flavonoïdes et pycnogénols," *International Journal for Vitamin and Nutrition Research* 49 (3) (1979): 307–311.

Meunier M-T et al., "Inhibition of angiotension I converting enzyme by flavanolic compounds: in vitro and in vivo studies," *Planta Medica* (1986): 12–15.

Porter LJ, "Structure and chemical properties of the condensed tannins," in RW Hemingway, ed., *Plant Polyphenols* (New York: Plenum Publishing Corporation, 1992).

Renaud S and de Logeril M, "Wine, alcohol, platelets and the French paradox for coronary heart disease," *Lancet* 339 (1992): 1523.

St. Leger AS, Cochrane AL, and Moore F, "Factors associated with cardiac mortality in developed countries with particular reference to the consumption of wine," *Lancet* 1 (1979): 1017–1020.

Singleton VL, "Grape and wine phenolics: background and prospects," in University of California–Davis, *Grape and Wine Centennial Symposium Proceedings* (1980): 215–227.

Tixier JM, Godeau G, Robert AM, and Hornebeck W, "Evidence by in vivo studies that binding of pycnogenols to elastin affects its rate of degradation by elastases," *Biochemical Pharmacology* 33 (24) (1984): 3933–3939.

Suggested Readings

Balch, James. F., and Phyllis A. Balch. *Prescription for Nutritional Healing*, 2nd ed. Garden City Park, NY: Avery Publishing Group, 1997.

Kandaswami, Chithan, and Dallas Clouatre. *The Health Benefits of Grapeseed*. New Canaan, CT: Keats Publishing, Inc., 1998.

Kandaswami, Chithan, and Richard A. Passwater. *Pycnogenol: The Super "Protector" Nutrient*. New Canaan, CT: Keats Publishing, Inc., 1994.

Krystosik, James D. *Pycnogenol: Nature's Prescription for Aging, Allergies . . . .* Garrettsville, OH: Good News Press, 1995.

Schwitters, Bert, and Jack Masquelier. *OPC in Practice*, 2nd ed. Rome, Italy: Alfa Omega Editrice, 1995.

Index